POSTPARTUM PILATES FOR WOMEN: A Path to A Renewed You

A Post Pregnancy Pilates Journey of Strength and Self-Discovery for Every Stage of Recovery

Dr Jessica McBerry

INTRODUCTION

Embark on a Journey of Postpartum Healing and Empowerment: Find Strength, Joy, and Confidence with Pilates

Welcome, mama, to this remarkable journey of rediscovering yourself after childbirth. Motherhood is a beautiful, transformative experience, yet it can also leave you feeling physically and emotionally depleted. The postpartum period is a time for healing, for nurturing your newborn, and for gently reclaiming your own well-being. But where do you begin?

This book is your guide to reclaiming your strength, joy, and confidence through the transformative power of

Pilates. More than just exercise, Pilates offers a holistic approach to postpartum recovery, empowering you to:

Gently rebuild your core strength: Diastasis recti, weakened abdominal muscles, and pelvic floor concerns are common after childbirth. This book provides safe and effective Pilates exercises specifically designed to address these challenges, helping you regain stability and control.

Relieve aches and pains: Back pain, fatigue, and joint discomfort can plague new mothers. Pilates offers gentle stretches and targeted exercises that can alleviate these issues, promoting flexibility and pain relief.

Boost your energy and mood: The postpartum period can be physically and emotionally demanding. This book equips you with Pilates routines that energize your body and uplift your spirit, leaving you feeling refreshed and revitalized.

Connect with your body: Pregnancy and childbirth can leave you feeling disconnected from your body. Pilates offers a mindful approach to movement, helping you rediscover your strength and resilience, and fostering a deeper sense of self-awareness and body confidence.

Find joy in movement: Exercise shouldn't feel like a chore. This book offers a playful and engaging approach to Pilates, with modifications and variations to suit your needs and fitness level, ensuring you find joy in every movement.

Whether you're a seasoned Pilates enthusiast or a complete beginner, this book is for you. It is your personal coach, your cheerleader, and your trusted companion on this journey of postpartum healing and rediscovery.

Inside these pages, you'll find:

- A comprehensive overview of Pilates principles and modifications for postpartum bodies.
- Safe and effective Pilates routines for every stage of postpartum recovery, from the early weeks to months beyond.

- Expert tips on diastasis recti, pelvic floor strengthening, and postpartum back pain management.
- Mindful breathing and relaxation techniques to combat stress and promote emotional well-being.

More than just a fitness manual, this book is a testament to the strength, resilience, and incredible capabilities of mothers. It is an invitation to embrace this transformative time, to move your body with intention, and to rediscover the joy of movement and self-care.

Take a deep breath, mama. You've got this. Let's embark on this incredible journey together, one Pilates pose at a time.

CHAPTER ONE

THE POSTPARTUM JOURNEY: A ROADMAP TO RECOVERY AND RENEWAL

Understanding the physical and emotional changes after childbirth

Giving birth is a life-changing experience, and the journey into motherhood brings with it a wave of physical and emotional changes. It's important to be prepared for these transformations, which can be both beautiful and challenging.

Physical Changes:

Uterus: The uterus, which has grown to accommodate your baby, will gradually shrink back to its pre-pregnancy size. This process, called involution, can cause cramping and bleeding (lochia).

Abdomen: Your abdominal muscles have stretched and separated to make room for your baby. This can lead to diastasis recti, a gap between the two halves of your rectus abdominis muscle.

Pelvic Floor: The pelvic floor muscles, which support your bladder, bowels, and uterus, have been stretched and weakened during pregnancy and childbirth. This can lead to incontinence, weakened sexual function, and pelvic pain.

Hormones: Your hormones, which were surging during pregnancy, plummet after childbirth. This can cause mood swings, fatigue, and difficulty sleeping. These are often referred to as the "baby blues" and usually resolve within a few days to a week.

Other changes: You may also experience hair loss, changes in skin tone, and weight fluctuations.

Emotional Changes:

Mood swings: The hormonal changes after childbirth can cause a roller coaster of emotions. You may feel happy, sad, anxious, or overwhelmed all in the same day. These mood swings are normal and usually temporary.

Baby blues: As mentioned earlier, most new mothers experience the "baby blues" in the first few days to a week after childbirth. This is a normal reaction to the hormonal and physical changes you're going through.

Postpartum depression (PPD): PPD is a serious mental health condition that affects about 1 in 10 women after childbirth. Symptoms of PPD can include persistent sadness, anxiety, loss of interest in activities you used to enjoy, and difficulty bonding with your baby. If you're experiencing any of these symptoms, it's important to seek professional help.

Bonding with your baby: It's normal if it takes time to feel a strong bond with your baby. Don't pressure yourself and trust that the bond will develop naturally over time.

Identity shift: Becoming a mother can be a significant identity shift. You may be adjusting to your new role and responsibilities, and it's important to allow yourself time to adjust.

Remember, every woman's experience is different. Some women may experience more physical and emotional changes than others. The important thing is to be patient with yourself and your body, and to reach out for support if you need it.

Here are some additional tips for coping with the physical and emotional changes after childbirth:

- Get plenty of rest.
- Eat a healthy diet.
- Exercise regularly, but start slowly and listen to your body.
- Join a support group or talk to other mothers about your experiences.
- Seek professional help if you're experiencing symptoms of PPD.

With time, patience, and support, you can adjust to the changes after childbirth and embrace your new life as a mother.

Setting realistic expectations for your postpartum journey

Transitioning into motherhood is a whirlwind of emotions, physical changes, and newfound responsibilities. It's easy to fall into the trap of romanticised portrayals or compare your experience to others, leading to disappointment and unnecessary stress. Setting realistic expectations for your postpartum journey is crucial for navigating this transformative time with grace and self-compassion.

Here are some key areas to consider:

Physical Recovery:

Healing takes time: Your body has undergone incredible changes, and it needs time to heal. Expect fatigue, discomfort, and slow progress. Remember, comparing your timeline to others is unproductive; everyone heals at their own pace.

Listen to your body: Don't push yourself too hard. Pay attention to your energy levels and adjust your activities accordingly. Rest when you need to, and don't feel guilty about taking things slow.

Postpartum recovery isn't always glamorous. Expect unexpected leaks, hormonal fluctuations, and unpredictable emotions. These are normal parts of the process, so don't let them define your experience.

Emotional Rollercoaster:

Baby blues are common: A rollercoaster of emotions is normal after childbirth. Accept the "baby blues" as a temporary hormonal shift and seek support if needed.

Bonding takes time: Don't pressure yourself to instantly feel a strong connection with your baby. The bond develops naturally through feeding, holding, and interaction. Trust the process and enjoy the journey.

New identity, new challenges: Embrace the changes in your identity and priorities. Motherhood brings new challenges and joys, so allow yourself to adapt and discover your new role.

Support and Self-care:

Seek support: Don't hesitate to ask for help. Lean on your partner, family, friends, and healthcare professionals. A strong support system is essential for your well-being.

Prioritize self-care: Make time for activities that nourish you, whether it's reading, taking a walk, or simply enjoying a quiet moment. Remember, taking care of yourself is not selfish; it's essential for being a good mother.

Celebrate small wins: Acknowledge and celebrate your progress, no matter how small. Every step forward is a victory in your postpartum journey.

Remember:

Every woman's experience is unique: Don't compare your journey to others. Focus on your own needs and celebrate your individual path to motherhood.

There's no shame in seeking help: If you're struggling, don't hesitate to reach out for professional help. You deserve to be supported and empowered during this significant transition.

By setting realistic expectations, practicing self-compassion, and embracing the support of others, you can navigate your postpartum journey with confidence and resilience. Remember, you are not alone in this, and you are capable of incredible strength and love.

The importance of self-care and listening to your body

In the whirlwind of new motherhood, prioritizing self-care and listening to your body can feel like a luxury, not a necessity. However, it's crucial for navigating the postpartum journey with grace and resilience. Here's why:

Why Self-Care Matters:

Reduces stress and anxiety: The postpartum period is naturally stressful, with hormonal fluctuations, sleep deprivation, and new responsibilities. Self-care activities like meditation, spending time in nature, or connecting with loved ones can help manage stress and improve mental well-being.

Boosts energy and resilience: Taking care of yourself physically and emotionally replenishes your energy reserves, making you better equipped to handle the demands of motherhood.

Improves mood and reduces depression: Self-care practices like exercise and healthy eating can positively impact your mood and reduce the risk of postpartum depression.

Strengthens relationships: When you take care of yourself, you're better equipped to nurture healthy relationships with your partner, baby, and others.

Listening to Your Body:

Physical cues: Pay attention to fatigue, soreness, or discomfort. These are your body's way of telling you to slow down or modify your activities. Pushing through can lead to injuries or hinder your recovery.

Emotional needs: Notice your emotional state. If you're feeling overwhelmed, anxious, or disconnected, find healthy ways to cope, like talking to a therapist or practicing relaxation techniques.

Intuition and gut feeling: Trust your intuition. If something feels wrong, don't ignore it. Listen to your inner voice and take steps to prioritize your needs.

How to Implement Self-Care and Body Listening:

Start small: Begin with manageable activities like taking a short walk, taking a warm bath, or reading a few pages of a book.

Schedule self-care time: Block time in your calendar for activities that nourish you, even if it's just 15 minutes a day.

Delegate and ask for help: Don't be afraid to ask for help with housework, childcare, or errands. Allow others to support you so you can focus on your well-being.

Connect with your body: Practice mindfulness exercises like yoga or meditation to tune into your body's sensations and needs.

Communicate openly: Talk to your partner, family, or healthcare professional about your needs and challenges. Open communication fosters support and understanding.

Remember: Self-care isn't selfish; it's essential. By prioritizing your well-being, you're not only taking care of yourself, but also creating a stronger foundation for caring for your baby and navigating the joys and challenges of motherhood. Listen to your body, embrace self-care as a non-negotiable, and watch your confidence and resilience blossom.

CHAPTER TWO

THE POWER OF PILATES: A HOLISTIC APPROACH TO POSTPARTUM FITNESS

Navigating the postpartum journey requires intentional choices to support your body's healing and emotional well-being. Enter Pilates, a gentle yet effective exercise method that shines when it comes to postpartum recovery. Here's why:

Physical Benefits:

Safe and Low-Impact: Unlike high-impact workouts, Pilates focuses on controlled movements and mindful breathing, minimizing stress on your joints and recovering muscles.

Strengthens Core and Pelvic Floor: Pilates targets your deep core muscles, promoting abdominal muscle reconnection and pelvic floor strengthening, crucial for diastasis recti and incontinence prevention.

Improves Posture and Flexibility: Pregnancy and childbirth can lead to postural imbalances. Pilates helps you regain proper alignment, reduce back pain, and improve overall flexibility.

Boosts Energy and Reduces Fatigue: Regular Pilates practice can improve circulation and oxygen flow, leading to increased energy levels and reduced postpartum fatigue.

Gentle Weight Management: Pilates helps build lean muscle mass, which can support healthy weight management and postpartum body confidence.

Mental and Emotional Benefits:

Stress Reduction and Relaxation: Pilates incorporates mindful breathing and focused movements, promoting stress reduction and anxiety management, common postpartum challenges.

Body Awareness and Mindfulness: Pilates helps you reconnect with your body and its sensations, fostering a sense of self-awareness and body appreciation.

Improves Mood and Self-Confidence: Regular exercise releases endorphins, natural mood boosters, combating postpartum blues and promoting positive well-being.

Social Connection and Community: Group Pilates classes can provide a supportive environment for connecting with other mothers, reducing isolation and fostering a sense of community.

Additional Advantages:

Modifiable for Different Levels: Pilates exercises can be adapted for various fitness levels and postpartum stages, ensuring a safe and effective workout for everyone.

Scalable at Home: Many Pilates routines can be practiced at home with minimal equipment, offering convenient and accessible exercise options.

Complements Other Therapies: Pilates can complement other postpartum therapies like physical therapy or massage, providing a holistic approach to recovery.

Remember, Always consult your healthcare professional before starting any new exercise program, especially after childbirth.

In conclusion, Pilates offers a wealth of benefits for postpartum recovery. Its gentle nature, focus on core and pelvic floor strength, and emphasis on mindfulness make it an ideal choice for new mothers seeking to rebuild their physical and emotional well-being. Embrace Pilates as a tool for healing, empowerment, and rediscovering your strength and confidence in this transformative time.

The benefits of Pilates for physical and mental well-being

Pilates is a mind-body exercise method that combines controlled movements, precise breathing, and mental focus. It's often associated with graceful movements and core strength, but its benefits extend far beyond just that. Here's a look at how Pilates can positively impact both your physical and mental well-being:

Physical Benefits:

Improved posture and alignment: Pilates emphasizes proper alignment throughout your movements, which can help correct imbalances and prevent pain. Imagine standing tall with your shoulders back and core engaged, like this:

Increased flexibility and range of motion: Pilates helps lengthen and loosen muscles, improving your overall flexibility and range of motion, making you feel more limber and agile. Think of effortlessly reaching for something on a high shelf.

Stronger core and pelvic floor: Pilates specifically targets your core and pelvic floor muscles, which are crucial for stability, back support, and preventing issues like incontinence. Imagine a strong foundation holding everything together, just like this:

Reduced pain and discomfort: Pilates can help alleviate chronic pain, especially in the back and joints, by improving posture, strengthening muscles, and promoting proper movement patterns.

Improved balance and coordination: Pilates exercises challenge your balance and coordination, making you feel more stable and confident in your movements. Imagine walking confidently on uneven terrain.

Weight management and body composition: While not solely focused on weight loss, Pilates can help build lean muscle mass, which increases your metabolism and aids in healthy weight management.

Mental Benefits:

Reduced stress and anxiety: The controlled movements and focus on breathing in Pilates can activate the parasympathetic nervous system, promoting relaxation and reducing stress and anxiety. Imagine taking a deep breath and feeling your worries melt away.

Improved mood and well-being: Pilates releases endorphins, natural mood boosters, which can elevate your mood and combat symptoms of depression. Imagine feeling a wave of happiness after a good workout.

Increased self-awareness and mindfulness: Pilates emphasizes connecting your mind and body, improving your awareness of your posture, movements, and sensations. Imagine feeling more in tune with your body and present in the moment.

Enhanced focus and concentration: The focus and precision required in Pilates can translate into improved concentration and focus in other areas of your life.

Imagine being able to tackle tasks with laser-sharp attention.

Greater confidence and self-esteem: As you see your physical and mental strength improve through Pilates, your confidence and self-esteem will naturally rise. Imagine feeling empowered and capable in your own skin.

Pilates offers a unique blend of physical and mental benefits, making it a valuable tool for anyone seeking to improve their overall well-being. Whether you're a seasoned athlete or just starting out, Pilates can be adapted to your individual needs and fitness level. So, why not give it a try and experience the transformative power of Pilates for yourself?

Remember, consistency is key to reaping the full benefits of Pilates. Aim for at least 2-3 sessions per week and gradually increase the intensity as you get stronger. With dedication and practice, you'll be amazed at how Pilates can enhance your physical and mental well-being, leaving you feeling stronger, happier, and more confident in your own skin.

Debunking myths and misconceptions about Pilates

Pilates, with its graceful movements and focus on core strength, has gained popularity in recent years. However, several myths and misconceptions surround this effective exercise method. Let's debunk some of the most common ones:

- **Myth #1: Pilates is only for women.**

Fact: Pilates is for everyone, regardless of gender, age, or fitness level. Men and women can benefit equally from its focus on building strength, flexibility, and balance.

- **Myth #2: Pilates is just stretching.**

Fact: While Pilates incorporates stretching, it also involves controlled movements that target various muscle groups, particularly your core. This builds strength, improves posture, and enhances overall body awareness.

- **Myth #3: Pilates is only for the flexible.**

Fact: You don't need to be a contortionist to do Pilates! Exercises can be modified to accommodate different levels of flexibility. As you progress, your flexibility will naturally improve.

- **Myth #4: Pilates is boring and not a real workout.**

Fact: Don't underestimate Pilates! While the movements may appear gentle, they engage your muscles deeply, leading to an effective workout that can be surprisingly challenging. You'll feel the burn, but in a good way!

- **Myth #5: You need expensive equipment to do Pilates.**

Fact: While specialized equipment like reformers and cadillac chairs exist, Pilates can be done effectively with minimal equipment, or even bodyweight exercises. You can easily find beginner routines online or attend mat Pilates classes that require no equipment at all.

- **Myth #6: Pilates is dangerous for pregnant women.**

Fact: When modified appropriately, Pilates can be a safe and beneficial exercise program for pregnant women. It can help strengthen core muscles, improve posture, and prepare the body for childbirth. However, it's crucial to consult your doctor before starting any new exercise program during pregnancy.

- **Myth #7: Pilates is just a fad.**

Fact: Pilates has been around for over a century and continues to grow in popularity worldwide. Its effectiveness and versatility have cemented its place as a valuable tool for improving physical and mental well-being.

So, the next time you hear a negative stereotype about Pilates, remember these debunked myths! Give it a try and experience the amazing benefits this exercise method has to offer for yourself.

CHAPTER THREE

Releasing Tension and Realigning Your Core

Exercises to safely engage and strengthen your abdominal muscles

Engaging and strengthening your abdominal muscles after childbirth is crucial for regaining core stability, preventing diastasis recti, and improving overall posture. Here are some safe and effective exercises to get you started:

Gentle Core Engagement:

Pelvic tilts: Lie on your back with knees bent and feet flat on the floor.

Engage your core by drawing your navel towards your spine, tilting your pelvis slightly. Hold for 5 seconds, then relax. Repeat 10-12 times.

Diaphragmatic breathing: Lie on your back with one hand on your chest and the other on your abdomen. Breathe deeply, feeling your abdomen rise and fall with each breath. This activates your diaphragm and deep core muscles. Practice for 5-10 minutes daily.

Bird-dog: Start on all fours, hands shoulder-width apart and knees hip-width apart. Keep your back flat and core engaged. Extend one arm forward and the opposite leg back, keeping your spine and hips stable.

Hold for a few seconds, then return to the starting position. Repeat on the other side. Do 10-12 repetitions per side.

Progressive Core Strengthening:

Dead bug: Lie on your back with knees bent and feet flat on the floor. Extend one arm straight overhead and the opposite leg straight out behind you. Engage your core and lower your arm and leg until they are just hovering off the floor. Hold for a few seconds, then return to the starting position. Repeat on the other side. Do 10-12 repetitions per side.

Side plank variations: Start in a side plank with your elbow directly below your shoulder and feet stacked or staggered. Hold for 30 seconds to a minute on each side. Progress to variations like raising your top leg or adding arm movements.

Hollow hold: Lie on your back and press your lower back into the floor. Engage your core and lift your legs and shoulders off the ground, keeping your body straight. Hold for as long as you can comfortably, aiming for 30 seconds initially.

Always remember:

- Listen to your body and stop if you feel any pain.
- Start with gentle exercises and gradually progress as you get stronger.

- Breathe deeply and control throughout each exercise.
- Maintain proper form and avoid overexertion.
- Consult your healthcare professional before starting any new exercise program, especially after childbirth.

These are just a few examples, and there are many other safe and effective exercises to strengthen your abdominal muscles. Feel free to research and find variations that work best for you. With consistent practice and proper form, you can safely engage and strengthen your core muscles, leading to better posture, improved balance, and a stronger, healthier you.

Techniques for improving posture and alleviating back pain

Good posture doesn't just look good, it also feels good and can significantly reduce back pain. Here are some effective techniques you can incorporate into your daily routine to improve your posture and alleviate back pain:

Stretching and Strengthening:

Cat-Cow: This gentle yoga pose stretches and strengthens your back muscles. Start on all fours with your hands shoulder-width apart and knees hip-width apart. Inhale as you arch your back and look up (cow), then exhale as you round your back and tuck your chin (cat). Repeat 10-12 times.

Child's Pose: This relaxing pose helps lengthen your spine and relieve tension in your lower back. Kneel on the floor with your toes together and sit back on your heels. Rest your forehead on the floor and extend your arms out in front of you. Hold for 5-10 minutes.

Chest Opener: This stretch helps open up your chest and improve your posture. Stand with your feet shoulder-width apart and arms bent at 90 degrees with elbows pointing towards the floor. Clasp your hands behind your back and gently push your chest forward, keeping your shoulders down. Hold for 30 seconds to a minute.

Strengthening Exercises:

Plank: This exercise strengthens your core muscles, which support your spine and improve posture. Start on all fours with your hands shoulder-width apart and elbows directly below your shoulders. Extend your legs back into a straight plank position. Hold for 30 seconds to a minute, as long as you can maintain good form.

Side Plank: This variation of the plank targets your obliques and helps improve your balance and stability. Start in a side plank position with your elbow directly below your shoulder and feet stacked or staggered. Hold for 30 seconds to a minute on each side.

Superman: This exercise strengthens your back muscles and improves posture. Lie on your stomach with your arms and legs extended. Lift your head, chest, arms, and legs off the ground as much as you can, keeping your core engaged. Hold for a few seconds, then lower back down. Repeat 10-12 times.

Some Posture Tips:

Stand tall: Imagine a string pulling you up from the crown of your head. Keep your shoulders back and down, and your chin slightly tucked in.

Sit up straight:When sitting, avoid slouching and keep your back straight against the chair. Your knees should be bent at 90 degrees and your feet flat on the floor.

Mind your desk setup: Adjust your computer screen to eye level and ensure your chair provides good back support. Take frequent breaks to stand up and move around.

Stretch throughout the day: Don't let your muscles get tight! Take short breaks to stretch your back, neck, and shoulders throughout the day.

Wear supportive shoes: Choose shoes that fit well and provide good arch support. Avoid wearing high heels for extended periods.

Extra Tips:

Maintain a healthy weight: Excess weight can put strain on your back and lead to pain.

Stay hydrated: Drinking plenty of water helps keep your spine discs lubricated and healthy.

Manage stress: Stress can contribute to back pain. Practice relaxation techniques like yoga or meditation to manage stress levels.

Seek professional help: If your back pain is severe or persistent, consult a healthcare professional for diagnosis and treatment.

Remember, improving posture and alleviating back pain is a process. Be patient, consistent with your efforts, and you'll gradually see and feel the results. A healthy body starts with a strong foundation, and good posture is key to achieving that.

Breathing Exercises for Relaxation and Stress Management

Taking a deep breath is a simple yet powerful way to calm your mind, reduce stress, and improve your overall well-being. Here are three effective breathing exercises you can practice anytime, anywhere:

- 1. **Diaphragmatic Breathing:**

This fundamental technique engages your diaphragm, the primary muscle of respiration, leading to deeper and more efficient breaths.

How to do it:
Lie down or sit comfortably with your back straight. Place one hand on your chest and the other on your stomach. Breathe in slowly through your nose, feeling your stomach expand outward. Breathe out slowly through pursed lips, feeling your stomach draw inwards. Focus on feeling the movement of your diaphragm with each breath. Repeat for 5-10 minutes.

- **2.   Alternate   Nostril Breathing:**

This ancient practice, also known as Nadi Shodhana, balances the flow of energy in your body, promoting relaxation and focus.

How to do it:
Sit comfortably with your back straight and close your eyes. Raise your right hand and gently touch your right nostril with your thumb and your left nostril with your ring finger. Inhale slowly through your left nostril, close your left nostril with your ring finger, and exhale slowly through your right nostril. Repeat the inhale through the right nostril, exhale through the left, for 5-10 minutes.

3. 4-7-8 Breathing:

This technique, popularized by Dr. Andrew Weil, combines rhythmic breathing with visualization to calm the nervous system and promote relaxation.

How to do it:

Sit comfortably with your back straight and close your eyes. Exhale completely through your mouth, making a whooshing sound. Inhale slowly through your nose for a count of 4. Hold your breath for a count of 7. Exhale slowly through your mouth for a count of 8, making the whooshing sound again. Repeat the cycle for 4-7 breaths.

Remember:

- Breathe deeply and rhythmically.

- Focus on your breath and feel the movement of your diaphragm.
- Practice regularly for optimal results.
- If you have any underlying health conditions, consult your doctor before starting any new breathing exercises.

These are just a few examples, and many other breathing exercises can help you relax and manage stress. Experiment with different techniques and find what works best for you. With consistent practice, you can harness the power of your breath to cultivate inner peace and well-being.

Here are some additional tips for effective breathing exercises:

- Find a quiet and comfortable place to practice.
- Close your eyes or focus on a soft spot to minimize distractions.
- Wear loose-fitting clothing that doesn't restrict your breathing.
- Be gentle with yourself and don't force your breath.
- Enjoy the process and allow yourself to relax.

May your breath be your guide to a calmer and more balanced you!

CHAPTER FOUR

Building Pelvic Floor Strength and Confidence

The pelvic floor, a group of muscles and connective tissues at the base of the pelvis, plays a crucial role in postpartum recovery. During pregnancy and childbirth, these muscles undergo significant changes, stretching and weakening to accommodate the growing baby and delivery. This can lead to various challenges, including:

Pelvic Floor Dysfunction: This encompasses a range of issues like urinary incontinence (leakage), fecal incontinence, pelvic organ prolapse (bulging of organs), and sexual dysfunction.

Diastasis Recti: Separation of the abdominal muscles, which can affect core strength and contribute to back pain.

Pain and discomfort: Weakened pelvic floor muscles can contribute to pain in the pelvic area, back, and legs.

Loss of sensation: Some women experience decreased sensation in the vaginal area after childbirth.

However, the good news is that with proper care and rehabilitation, the pelvic floor can bounce back remarkably. Understanding its role in recovery empowers you to take proactive steps towards a healthy and comfortable life after childbirth.

Here's how the pelvic floor helps in postpartum recovery:

1. Supports Organs: The pelvic floor acts as a hammock, supporting the bladder, uterus, rectum, and small intestine. Strong pelvic floor muscles prevent these organs from prolapsing, leading to better bladder and bowel control.

2. Improves Core Stability: A strong pelvic floor works in synergy with abdominal muscles to provide core stability and support. This improves posture, reduces back pain, and aids in lifting and carrying.

3. Enhances Sexual Function: The pelvic floor plays a vital role in sexual pleasure and arousal. Strengthening these muscles can improve sensitivity, orgasm intensity, and overall sexual satisfaction.

4. Promotes Healing: Pelvic floor exercises can improve blood flow to the area, enhancing tissue healing and reducing pain after childbirth.

5. Prevents Future Issues: Addressing pelvic floor weakness early on can prevent the development of long-term complications like urinary incontinence or prolapse.

So, what can you do to support your pelvic floor in postpartum recovery?

1. Pelvic Floor Exercises: Kegels are the most well-known exercises, but there are many other options to target different aspects of pelvic floor function. Consult a physiotherapist or healthcare professional for personalized guidance.

2. Awareness and Activation: Pay attention to your pelvic floor throughout the day. Engage and lift it during activities like coughing, sneezing, or lifting.

3. Healthy Habits: Maintain a healthy weight, stay hydrated, and avoid constipation to reduce pressure on the pelvic floor.

4. Listen to Your Body: Don't push yourself too hard. Rest when needed, and prioritize activities that feel comfortable and enjoyable.

5. Seek Support: Don't hesitate to seek help from a healthcare professional if you experience any concerns about your pelvic floor function.

Remember, recovery is a journey, not a race. Be patient with yourself, celebrate your progress, and empower your pelvic floor to be the powerhouse it truly is. With dedication and the right guidance, you can pave the way for a healthy and fulfilling life after childbirth.

Gentle Exercises to Improve Pelvic Floor Tone and Prevent Incontinence

Strengthening your pelvic floor muscles is crucial after childbirth and for overall bladder control. Here are some gentle exercises you can do at home to improve tone and prevent incontinence:

1. Kegels:

The classic! Squeeze your pelvic floor as if you're trying to stop a flow of urine. Hold for 5 seconds, then relax for 5 seconds. Repeat 10-15 times, 3-4 sets per day.

2. Pelvic Floor Lifts:

Lie on your back with knees bent and feet flat on the floor. Engage and lift your pelvic floor as if pulling it upwards. Hold for 5 seconds, then relax. Repeat 10-15 times, 3-4 sets per day.

3. Heel Slides:

Sit on a chair with your back straight and feet flat on the floor. Slide your heels forward on the floor as you engage your pelvic floor, then slide them back while relaxing. Repeat 10-15 times, 3-4 sets per day.

4. Bridge:

Lie on your back with knees bent and feet flat on the floor. Press your heels into the ground and lift your hips off the floor, squeezing your glutes and pelvic floor. Hold for 5 seconds, then lower back down. Repeat 10-15 times, 3-4 sets per day.

5. Cat-Cow:

Start on all fours with your hands shoulder-width apart and knees hip-width apart. Inhale and arch your back, looking up (cow). Exhale and round your back, tucking your chin (cat). Repeat 10 times.

Remember:

- Start slowly and gradually increase the duration and intensity of your exercises.
- Breathe deeply and control throughout the exercises.
- Focus on engaging your pelvic floor muscles, not just contracting your abdominal muscles.
- Stop if you experience any pain or discomfort.
- If you have any concerns or questions, consult your healthcare professional.

Additional Tips:

- Practice good posture throughout the day to engage your pelvic floor passively.
- Stay hydrated to maintain proper bladder function.
- Avoid heavy lifting and straining to prevent putting pressure on your pelvic floor.
- Consider wearing supportive clothing, like pelvic floor-specific underwear, for added support.

These gentle exercises can be easily incorporated into your daily routine and can make a significant difference in improving your pelvic floor tone and preventing incontinence. Remember, consistency is key, so make it a habit and celebrate your progress along the way!

For further guidance and personalized exercises, consult a pelvic floor physiotherapist.** They can assess your individual needs and recommend the most effective exercises for you.

Tips for managing diastasis recti and other common postpartum issues

Diastasis recti, along with other common postpartum issues like pelvic floor dysfunction and back pain, can be daunting after childbirth. But fear not, mama! By prioritizing self-care and implementing some key strategies, you can manage these challenges and pave the way for a healthy and fulfilling journey back to yourself. Here are some helpful tips:

Managing Diastasis Recti:

Gentle exercise: Avoid traditional crunches and high-impact workouts that strain your abdominal muscles. Opt for low-impact exercises like pelvic floor lifts, modified planks, and side-lying leg raises.

Posture awareness: Maintain good posture throughout the day to prevent further separation. Engage your core while sitting, standing, and lifting.

Diastasis recti-specific exercises: Consult a physiotherapist or healthcare professional for personalized exercises that target the deep core muscles and promote abdominal wall closure.

Abdominal taping: While not a cure, therapeutic taping can offer temporary support and proprioceptive feedback.

Patience and consistency: Healing takes time. Be patient with your body and focus on gradual progress. Consistency is key, so incorporate these strategies into your daily routine.

Managing Pelvic Floor Dysfunction:

Pelvic floor exercises: Kegels are a classic, but there are many other exercises to target different aspects of pelvic floor function. Consult a physiotherapist or healthcare professional for personalized guidance.

Bladder retraining: If you experience incontinence, practice holding and releasing urine in controlled intervals to strengthen your pelvic floor and bladder control.

Healthy habits: Maintain a healthy weight, stay hydrated, and avoid constipation to reduce pressure on the pelvic floor.

Seek professional help: If you have concerns or persistent issues, don't hesitate to seek help from a physiotherapist or healthcare professional.

Managing Back Pain:

Posture awareness: Maintain good posture throughout the day to prevent strain on your back muscles.

Gentle stretches and strengthening exercises: Focus on exercises that target your core and back muscles, like bridges, bird-dogs, and side planks.

Ergonomics: Pay attention to your posture while sitting, standing, and carrying your baby. Use supportive cushions and chairs.

Warmth and massage: Applying heat pads or getting a massage can help relax tight muscles and relieve pain.

Listen to your body: Avoid activities that aggravate your pain and take breaks when needed.

General Tips for Postpartum Recovery:

Prioritize rest and relaxation: Your body needs time to heal. Listen to your fatigue cues and prioritize sleep and relaxation.

Healthy eating and hydration: Nourish your body with nutrient-rich foods and stay hydrated to support healing and energy levels.

Seek support: Don't hesitate to ask for help from your partner, family, friends, or healthcare professionals.

Connect with other moms: Sharing experiences and advice with other mothers can be invaluable.

Mental and emotional well-being: Practice self-care activities you enjoy, like meditation, yoga, or spending time in nature.

Celebrate your progress: Focus on how far you've come, not how far you have to go. Celebrate each small victory on your journey to recovery.

Remember, every woman's postpartum experience is unique. These tips are a starting point, and you may need to adjust them based on your individual needs and recovery pace. Consult your healthcare professional for personalised guidance and support.

With patience, self-care, and the right strategies, you can manage common postpartum issues and embrace a healthy and fulfilling journey into motherhood. You've got this, mama!

CHAPTER FIVE

FINDING STABILITY AND BALANCE IN YOUR CORE

Regaining your balance and coordination after childbirth is crucial for staying active, confident, and preventing falls. Here are some effective and safe exercises to get you back on your feet:

Gentle Movements:

Heel-toe walking: Walk heel-to-toe in a straight line, focusing on precise foot placement and maintaining good posture. This improves balance and coordination while engaging your core.

Side-stepping: Take small side steps, alternating your feet, while keeping your core engaged and body stable. This challenges your balance and strengthens your lateral muscles.

Tandem walking: Place one foot directly in front of the other, heel-to-toe, and walk forward slowly. This activates your core and ankle stability.

Strengthening Exercises:

Single-leg balance: Stand on one leg for as long as you can comfortably hold, then switch to the other leg. This strengthens your core, ankles, and leg muscles, improving overall balance.

Chair squats: Sit and stand from a chair slowly and controlled, focusing on engaging your core and leg muscles. This strengthens your lower body and improves balance when rising from a seated position.

Plank variations: Start on your forearms or hands in a plank position, hold for 30 seconds to a minute, and gradually increase the duration. You can also try side planks or planks with leg lifts for added challenge.

COORDINATION ACTIVITIES:

Ball toss and catch: Toss a small ball up and down with one hand, then switch hands. This improves hand-eye coordination and reaction time.

Ball dribbling: Dribble a small ball around cones or obstacles, using both feet and focusing on agility and coordination.

Dance or movement classes: Joining a dance or fitness class specifically designed for postpartum recovery can be a fun and effective way to improve your balance and coordination in a supportive environment.

Remember:

- Start with gentle exercises and gradually increase the intensity as you get stronger.
- Focus on proper form and technique to avoid injuries.

- Listen to your body and stop if you experience any pain or discomfort.
- Consult your healthcare professional before starting any new exercise program, especially after childbirth.

These are just a few examples, and there are many other exercises you can do to improve your balance and coordination. Explore different options, find what you enjoy, and make it a part of your regular routine. With consistent practice and the right approach, you'll be back on your feet feeling confident and balanced in no time!

Additionally, consider incorporating activities like yoga, tai chi, or Pilates, which emphasize body awareness and balance. Remember, the key is to find activities you enjoy and that fit your fitness level and recovery needs. Embrace the journey, celebrate your progress, and enjoy regaining your balance and confidence after childbirth!

Techniques for regaining strength and control over your movements

Regaining strength and control over your movements after childbirth requires a multi-faceted approach. Here are some techniques you can incorporate to achieve this goal:

Gradual Strength Training:

Focus on core and pelvic floor: Engage your core muscles in everyday activities like sit-ups, squats, and lunges. Invest in pelvic floor exercises like Kegels to strengthen your pelvic floor muscles, improving bladder control and preventing prolapse.

Low-impact exercises: Gentle exercises like swimming, yoga, Pilates, or walking are excellent for rebuilding strength without putting excessive strain on your body.

Progressive overload: Gradually increase the difficulty of your exercises by adding weight, sets, or reps as your strength improves.

Body Awareness and Proprioception:

Mindful movement: Pay attention to your body's sensations and movements during exercise and daily activities. This enhances your awareness of your body and how it moves in space.

Balance exercises: Activities like single-leg stands, tai chi, or wobble boards challenge your balance and improve your ability to control your movements in different situations.

Sensory integration: Activities like yoga or dancing can help you reconnect with your senses and integrate them into your movement patterns, leading to greater control and coordination.

Rest and Recovery:

Listen to your body: Don't push yourself too hard. Take rest days when needed and prioritize sleep to allow your muscles and body to recover properly.

Hydration and nutrition: Stay hydrated and nourish your body with nutrient-rich foods to support muscle repair and energy levels.

Stress management: Chronic stress can hinder recovery. Practice stress-management techniques like meditation, deep breathing, or spending time in nature to promote overall well-being.

Additional Techniques:

Seek professional guidance: Consult a physiotherapist or healthcare professional for personalized exercise plans and guidance tailored to your specific needs and recovery stage.

Warm-up and cool-down: Always warm up before exercise and cool down afterwards to prepare your muscles and prevent injuries.

Listen to your intuition: If something feels wrong, stop and reassess. Trust your body's signals and adjust your activities accordingly.

Remember, regaining strength and control over your movements takes time and dedication. Be patient with yourself, celebrate your progress, and enjoy the journey back to feeling empowered and confident in your body.

With the right approach and a combination of these techniques, you can confidently reclaim your strength and control over your movements after childbirth, embracing a stronger and more empowered you.

Finding your center and building a strong foundation for future activities

Finding your center and building a strong foundation isn't just a physical pursuit, it's a holistic journey encompassing your mind, body, and spirit. Here are some steps to guide you:

Physical Foundation:

Body awareness: Practice mindfulness and connect with your physical sensations. Pay attention to your breath, posture, and movement. Activities like yoga, meditation, or somatic movement can be helpful.

Core strength: Develop a strong core that supports your entire body. Include exercises like planks, bridges, and Pilates in your routine.

Balance and coordination: Challenge yourself with activities like single-leg stands, tai chi, or dance. Improving these skills will enhance your overall stability and control.

Healthy habits: Prioritize sleep, hydration, and a nutrient-rich diet to fuel your body and optimize its performance.

Mental Center:

Mindfulness and meditation: Cultivate present-moment awareness through practices like meditation or mindful breathing. This helps you quiet internal chatter and find inner peace.

Positive affirmations: Repeat positive statements that resonate with you to boost your confidence and self-belief.

Gratitude practice: Focus on the things you are grateful for, even the small things. This fosters a positive outlook and strengthens your inner foundation.

Journaling: Reflecting on your thoughts and emotions can help you gain clarity and identify areas for growth.

Spiritual Connection:

Explore your values: What matters most to you? Identifying your core values can guide your decisions and actions.

Connect with nature: Spend time in nature, immerse yourself in its beauty, and feel its grounding energy.

Engage in activities that nourish your soul: Whether it's art, music, spending time with loved ones, or pursuing a passion, prioritize activities that bring you joy and fulfillment.

Building a Strong Foundation:
Consistency: Integrate these practices into your daily routine, even if it's just for a few minutes each day.

Patience and self-compassion: Be patient with yourself, setbacks are part of the process. Embrace them as opportunities to learn and grow.

Celebrate your progress: Acknowledge your achievements, no matter how small. This reinforces positive habits and motivates you to keep going.

Seek support: Surround yourself with supportive people who uplift and inspire you.

Finding your center and building a strong foundation is a lifelong journey. It's about continually learning, evolving, and prioritizing your well-being. By incorporating these practices into your life, you can create a solid base of physical, mental, and spiritual strength, empowering you to face future activities with confidence and clarity.

Remember, your center is unique to you. Explore different practices, find what resonates with your soul, and build a foundation that supports your individual growth and fulfillment.

CHAPTER SIX

Nurturing Your Body and Mind

Integrating mindfulness practices into your Pilates routine

Integrating mindfulness into your Pilates routine can be a transformative experience, taking you beyond physical exercise and into a deeper realm of self-awareness and connection. Here are some ways to weave mindfulness into your practice:

Before the Practice:

Set an intention: Before you begin, take a moment to set an intention for your practice. What do you hope to achieve? This could be anything from finding inner peace to improving your focus or strengthening your body.

Mindful breathing: Start with a few minutes of focused breathing. Sit or stand comfortably and observe your breath, without trying to control it. Notice the rise and fall of your chest and abdomen, the rhythm of your breath.

Body scan: Gently bring your attention to different parts of your body, starting with your toes and moving upwards. Notice any sensations, tensions, or areas of discomfort without judgment.

During the Movements:

Focus on the present moment: Pay close attention to your body as you move. Feel the muscles engage, the breath in your lungs, the contact of your feet with the mat. Avoid getting lost in thoughts about the past or future.

Synchronize breath with movement: Coordinate your breath with your Pilates movements. Exhale on exertion, inhale on expansion. This mindful connection creates a sense of flow and awareness.

Observe without judgment: Notice any thoughts or emotions that arise during your practice. Observe them without judgment and let them go.

Don't get caught up in any internal dialogue.

Appreciate the small details: Pay attention to the subtle sensations in your body, the feeling of your skin against the mat, the texture of the equipment. These small details can become anchors for your mindfulness practice.

After the Practice:

Meditate: Spend a few minutes in silent meditation after your practice. Allow your body and mind to settle, observe any lingering sensations or emotions.

Journaling: Reflect on your experience. What did you learn about yourself and your body? What did you find challenging or rewarding? Journaling can help you deepen your understanding of your practice.

Gratitude: Take a moment to express gratitude for your body, your health, and the opportunity to move and practice.

Additional Tips:

Start small: Begin by incorporating mindfulness into a few exercises during your routine. Gradually, you can extend it to your entire practice.

Be patient: Integrating mindfulness takes time and practice. Don't get discouraged if your mind wanders.

Gently bring your attention back to the present moment.

Explore different techniques: There are many ways to practice mindfulness. Experiment with different techniques like visualization, guided meditations, or mindful walking to find what resonates with you.

By integrating mindfulness into your Pilates routine, you can transform your practice into a holistic experience that nourishes your body, mind, and spirit. You'll develop a deeper connection with yourself, improve your focus and concentration, and move with greater grace and ease. So, take a breath, step onto your mat, and embark on a journey of mindful movement and self-discovery.

Techniques for managing stress and anxiety during the postpartum period

The postpartum period can be a whirlwind of emotions, with joy and excitement often accompanied by stress and anxiety. Here are some effective techniques you can use to manage these challenges and navigate this important time with greater peace and clarity:

Self-Care Practices:

Prioritize Sleep: Aim for 7-8 hours of sleep per night. Consider implementing sleep hygiene practices like setting a regular sleep schedule, creating a relaxing bedtime routine, and avoiding screens before bed.

Healthy Eating: Nourish your body with nutrient-rich foods that provide sustained energy and support your emotional well-being. Avoid sugary and processed foods that can worsen anxiety.

Exercise: Regular physical activity, even gentle walks or yoga, releases endorphins and reduces stress hormones. Find activities you enjoy and fit them into your routine.

Mindfulness and Relaxation: Practices like meditation, deep breathing exercises, or progressive muscle relaxation can help calm your mind and body. Dedicate a few minutes each day to quiet your mind and find inner peace.

Coping Strategies:

Identify Triggers: Pay attention to situations or thoughts that trigger your anxiety. Once identified, you can develop strategies to avoid or manage them effectively.

Challenge Negative Thoughts: Challenge negative self-talk and replace it with positive affirmations. Practice reframing your thoughts in a more realistic and helpful way.

Seek Support: Don't hesitate to reach out for support from your partner, family, friends, or a therapist.

Talking about your feelings and experiences can be incredibly helpful.

Join a Support Group: Connecting with other moms who understand what you're going through can be invaluable. Share your experiences, offer support to others, and feel empowered by the shared journey.

Additional Techniques:

Limit social media: Social media can be a breeding ground for comparison and negativity. Take breaks from platforms that trigger your anxiety and focus on real-world connections.

Delegate and ask for help: Don't be afraid to ask for help with household tasks, childcare, or errands. Delegating allows you to prioritize your own well-being.

Practice self-compassion: Be kind to yourself. Accept that this is a challenging time and allow yourself to feel your emotions. Celebrate your successes, big and small.

Seek professional help: If your stress or anxiety feels overwhelming or is impacting your daily life, don't hesitate to seek professional help from a therapist or counsellor.

Remember, managing stress and anxiety during the postpartum period is a journey, not a destination. Be patient with yourself, experiment with different techniques, and celebrate your progress along the way. You've got this, mama!

By taking care of yourself and implementing these techniques, you can navigate the postpartum period with greater resilience and emotional well-being, paving the way for a fulfilling and joyful journey into motherhood.

Cultivating self-compassion and body acceptance

Cultivating self-compassion and body acceptance is a beautiful and empowering journey towards a more fulfilling relationship with yourself. Here are some steps to guide you:

Self-Compassion:

Reframing negative self-talk: Notice and challenge the harsh inner critic within. Instead of judging yourself, rephrase those thoughts with kindness and understanding.

Mindful self-care: Prioritize activities that nourish your mind, body, and spirit. Listen to your needs and engage in practices like meditation, spending time in nature, or creative pursuits.

Acceptance and forgiveness: Accept that everyone makes mistakes and experiences challenges. Forgive yourself for past shortcomings and focus on learning and growth.

Gratitude practice: Take time each day to appreciate your body and its capabilities. Focus on the things you love about yourself, big or small.

Body Acceptance:

Challenge societal beauty standards: Recognize the unrealistic and harmful nature of mainstream beauty ideals. Choose to believe in your own unique beauty and worth.

Focus on health and well-being: Prioritize activities that make you feel good, not just look good. Nourish your body with healthy foods, engage in activities you enjoy, and celebrate your strength and resilience.

Positive affirmations: Repeat positive statements about your body that resonate with you. Focus on your strengths and qualities, not just physical appearance.

Mindful body scan: Practice mindful awareness of your body without judgment. Feel the sensations in different parts, acknowledge your strengths and areas you'd like to nurture, all with kindness and acceptance.

Additional Practices:

Surround yourself with supportive people: Choose friends and family who celebrate you for who you are, not just how you look.

Unfollow unrealistic accounts: Limit your exposure to media that promotes unrealistic beauty standards and focus on accounts that celebrate diversity and body positivity.

Celebrate small victories: Recognize and celebrate your progress, no matter how small. Every step towards self-compassion and body acceptance is a victory worth celebrating.

Seek professional help: If you struggle with negative body image or eating disorders, don't hesitate to seek professional help. A therapist can provide you with tools and support to overcome these challenges.

Remember, self-compassion and body acceptance are journeys, not destinations. There will be ups and downs, moments of doubt and progress. Be patient with yourself, celebrate your victories, and trust that you are worthy of love and acceptance, just as you are.

Embracing self-compassion and body acceptance is an empowering act of self-love. By prioritising your well-being, challenging harmful narratives, and celebrating your unique beauty, you pave the way for a more fulfilling and joyful relationship with yourself and your body.

CHAPTER SEVEN:

NOURISHING YOUR BODY FOR RECOVERY AND ENERGY

Importance of a healthy diet for postpartum healing and energy levels

A healthy diet plays a crucial role in postpartum healing and boosting your energy levels after childbirth. Here's why it's so important:

Replenishment and Repair:

Nutrient needs increase: Your body has been working hard during pregnancy and childbirth. It needs extra nutrients to repair tissues, rebuild blood volume, and support milk production if you're breastfeeding.

Essential vitamins and minerals: Vitamins like A, C, D, and B vitamins, along with minerals like iron, calcium, and magnesium, are vital for wound healing, immune function, and overall health.

Protein for tissue repair: Protein is essential for building and repairing tissues, from muscles to skin. Choose lean protein sources like fish, poultry, beans, and lentils.

Energy and Stamina:

Fuel your body: A balanced diet rich in complex carbohydrates, healthy fats, and protein provides sustained energy throughout the day. Avoid sugary foods that create energy crashes.

Hydration is key: Staying hydrated is vital for nutrient absorption and overall well-being. Aim for 8-10 glasses of water daily, and increase your intake if breastfeeding.

Fight fatigue: Iron deficiency is a common cause of fatigue in postpartum women. Include iron-rich foods like red meat, leafy greens, and lentils in your diet.

Mood and Emotional Well-being:

Gut health and brain health: A healthy gut microbiome is linked to improved mood and emotional well-being. Include probiotic-rich foods like yogurt, kimchi, and fermented vegetables in your diet.

Omega-3 fatty acids: These healthy fats support brain function and mood. Include fatty fish like salmon, tuna, and mackerel in your meals.

Reduce stress hormones: Certain foods like berries, dark chocolate, and nuts can help manage stress hormones and improve overall well-being.

Additional Tips:

Focus on whole foods: Prioritize whole, unprocessed foods like fruits, vegetables, whole grains, and lean protein sources. Limit sugary drinks, processed foods, and unhealthy fats.

Plan and prepare meals: Having healthy options readily available helps you make good choices, especially when time is tight.

Don't skip meals: Eating regular meals and snacks throughout the day helps maintain energy levels and prevents overeating later.

Seek professional guidance: If you have concerns about your diet or nutritional needs, talk to your doctor or a registered dietitian.

Remember, a healthy diet is not about deprivation, but about nourishing your body with the nutrients it needs to heal and thrive. Choose foods that make you feel good, experiment with different recipes, and find joy in nourishing yourself during this important time.

By prioritizing a healthy diet, you can support your body's healing journey, boost your energy levels, and feel your best as you navigate the joys and challenges of motherhood.

Tips for incorporating nutritious and delicious foods into your daily routine

Incorporating nutritious and delicious foods into your daily routine doesn't have to be a chore! Here are some tips to make it fun and sustainable:

Planning and Preparation:

Make a weekly meal plan: Plan your meals for the week, considering your schedule and preferences. This helps you avoid unhealthy choices when you're short on time.

Prep ingredients in advance: Wash, chop, and store fruits, vegetables, and grains ahead of time for easy access. This makes healthy snacking and quick meals a breeze.

Have healthy staples on hand: Stock your pantry with whole grains, lentils, beans, nuts, and seeds. These versatile ingredients can be used in countless dishes.

Cook in bulk: Prepare large batches of soups, stews, or roasted vegetables and portion them out for the week. This saves time and ensures you have healthy options readily available.

Incorporating Flavor and Variety:

Explore different cuisines: Experiment with recipes from diverse cultures. Try new spices, herbs, and cooking techniques to keep your meals exciting.

Focus on fresh ingredients: Seasonal fruits and vegetables offer the best flavor and nutrients. Visit farmers' markets or grow your own herbs for fresh additions.

Don't fear healthy fats: Healthy fats like avocado, olive oil, and nuts add richness and flavor to your meals.

Get creative with leftovers: Repurpose leftovers into new dishes. Leftover roasted vegetables can be added to salads or stir-fries, while cooked chicken can be used in sandwiches or wraps.

Embrace sweet treats: Enjoy naturally sweet fruits, dark chocolate, or homemade desserts made with whole ingredients.

Making it Convenient and Snack-able:

Pack healthy snacks: Keep pre-portioned fruits, nuts, yogurt, or veggie sticks in your bag for on-the-go snacking.

Make smoothies and dips: Blend fruits, vegetables, and yogurt for a nutritious and delicious beverage. Homemade dips with whole-grain crackers or veggies are a healthy alternative to store-bought snacks.

Involve the family: Get your family involved in meal planning and preparation. This makes it more fun and encourages everyone to eat healthier.

Remember:

Start small: Don't try to change everything overnight. Introduce one or two new healthy habits each week.

Be kind to yourself: Don't be discouraged by occasional slip-ups. Just get back on track with your next meal or snack.

Celebrate your successes: Acknowledge your progress and reward yourself for making healthy choices.

By incorporating these tips, you can make nutritious and delicious food a regular part of your daily routine. You'll feel better, have more energy, and discover a world of culinary delights along the way!

Staying hydrated and supporting your body's natural healing processes

Staying hydrated is crucial for overall health, but it takes on even greater importance during your body's natural healing processes, especially after childbirth. Here's why hydration is key and how to support your body's natural healing:

Why Hydration Matters:

Water makes up a large part of you: Around 60% of your adult body weight is water, and every cell, tissue, and organ needs it to function properly.

Hydration aids healing: Water transports nutrients to cells, helps flush out toxins, and lubricates joints, all essential for optimal healing.

Dehydration can hinder recovery: Dehydration can slow down wound healing, decrease energy levels, and contribute to fatigue, hindering your body's natural repair mechanisms.

Supporting Hydration:

Listen to your thirst: Don't wait until you're thirsty to drink. Aim to sip water throughout the day, even if you don't feel thirsty.

Choose water over sugary drinks: Sugary drinks can dehydrate you further and provide empty calories. Opt for plain water, herbal teas, or natural fruit-infused water.

Track your intake: Use a water bottle with markings or a hydration app to track your water intake throughout the day. Aim for 8-10 glasses of water daily, adjusting based on your activity level and climate.

Eat hydrating foods: Water-rich fruits and vegetables like watermelon, cucumber, and celery can contribute to your daily water intake.

Be mindful of caffeine and alcohol: These can be dehydrating, so moderate your intake and ensure you drink extra water if you consume them.

Additional Tips for Healing:

Prioritize rest and sleep: Your body needs time to heal. Aim for 7-8 hours of sleep each night and take naps when possible.

Nourish your body with a healthy diet: Choose nutritious foods rich in vitamins, minerals, and antioxidants to support your healing process.

Engage in gentle movement: Light exercise like walking or yoga can promote healing and improve circulation.

Manage stress: Chronic stress can hinder healing. Practice relaxation techniques like deep breathing or meditation to manage stress levels.

Seek support: Don't hesitate to reach out to your doctor or healthcare professional if you have any concerns about your healing process or hydration levels.

Remember, staying hydrated is a simple yet powerful way to support your body's natural healing abilities. By implementing these tips, you can give your body the optimal environment to recover and feel your best, both physically and emotionally.

By prioritizing hydration and incorporating these supportive practices, you can trust your body's natural healing mechanisms and embrace a journey towards renewed health and well-being.

SAMPLE PILATES ROUTINES FOR DIFFERENT STAGES OF POSTPARTUM RECOVERY

These are general guidelines, and it's crucial to consult your healthcare professional before starting any new exercise program, especially after childbirth. Listen to your body, modify as needed, and gradually increase intensity as you feel stronger.

EARLY POSTPARTUM (WEEKS 1-6):

Focus: Gentle movements to regain core engagement, improve mobility, and prevent diastasis recti.

Breathing exercises: Cat-cow, diaphragmatic breathing, and gentle side bending with breath.

Pelvic floor exercises: Kegels, pelvic tilts, and gentle leg lifts with pelvic floor engagement.

Modified Pilates poses: Modified planks on forearms or knees, supine leg circles, and side-lying leg lifts with controlled movements.

Relaxation: Incorporate gentle stretches and mindful breathing to promote healing and reduce stress.

MID-POSTPARTUM (WEEKS 6-12):

Focus: Gradually increase intensity, strengthen core and pelvic floor, and improve overall body control.

Standing Pilates exercises: Standing leg lifts, pelvic bridges, and controlled squats with good form.

Dynamic stretches: Arm circles, leg swings, and gentle lunges with controlled movements.

Pilates ball exercises: Modified Pilates exercises on a stability ball for an added challenge.

Core strengthening: Plank variations, dead bugs, and bird-dogs to target different aspects of your core.

LATE POSTPARTUM (WEEKS 12-24):

Focus: Rebuild strength, improve balance and coordination, and prepare for more vigorous activities.

Intermediate Pilates exercises: Regular planks, side planks, and abdominal roll-ups with proper form.

Balance and coordination exercises: Single-leg stances, controlled hops, and Pilates exercises with controlled rotations.

Cardio-Pilates: Combine Pilates movements with low-impact cardio like jumping jacks or jumping squats for an elevated heart rate.

Strengthening exercises: Squats with weights, lunges with weights, and upper-body exercises with light weights to build overall strength.

Additional Tips:

- Start with shorter routines (15-20 minutes) and gradually increase duration as you get stronger.

- Listen to your body and modify or stop any exercise that causes pain or discomfort.

- Warm up before and cool down after your workout.

- Stay hydrated throughout your workout.

- Don't be afraid to modify exercises to fit your needs and abilities.

- Enjoy the process and celebrate your progress!

Remember, these are just examples, and there are countless Pilates exercises and modifications available. Consult a certified Pilates instructor or healthcare professional for a personalized program tailored to your specific needs and goals. Have fun, listen to your body, and enjoy the journey back to your pre-pregnancy strength and well-being!

MODIFICATIONS FOR COMMON POSTPARTUM CONDITIONS

Here are some modifications for common postpartum conditions you might encounter while exercising:

Diastasis Recti:

- Avoid exercises that strain the abdominal wall, like full planks, crunches, and sit-ups.

- Focus on gentle core engagement exercises like pelvic tilts, side-lying leg lifts, and modified planks on forearms.

- Prioritize pelvic floor exercises like Kegels and bridges to support abdominal wall stability.

- Use modifications like performing exercises with knees bent or placing a small ball between your abdominal wall to avoid excessive strain.

- Consult a healthcare professional for personalized guidance and exercises specific to your diastasis recti severity.

Pelvic Floor Weakness:

- Start with gentle pelvic floor exercises like Kegels, focusing on proper contraction and relaxation.

- Progress to more challenging exercises like pelvic floor holds and bridges, ensuring proper form and avoiding straining.

- Avoid high-impact activities like jumping or running until your pelvic floor is sufficiently strengthened.

- Incorporate exercises that engage the core and pelvic floor together, like modified planks and side-lying leg lifts with pelvic floor engagement.

- Seek guidance from a pelvic floor therapist who can assess your individual needs and provide targeted exercises.

Episiotomy or C-Section:

- Focus on low-impact exercises that don't strain your incision or put pressure on your abdominal wall.

- Choose exercises that promote healing and circulation, like gentle walking, swimming, or yoga.

- Avoid strenuous activities like lifting heavy weights or exercises that involve jumping or twisting until your doctor clears you.

- Listen to your body and rest when needed. Healing takes time, so be patient and prioritize recovery.

- Consult your doctor before starting any new exercise program to ensure it's safe for your specific situation.

Postpartum Back Pain:

- Avoid exercises that strain your back, like deep backbends or twisting movements.

- Focus on gentle stretching and strengthening exercises for your core and back, like modified cat-cows, side planks, and bridges.

- Maintain proper posture during all exercises, engaging your core and avoiding slouching.

- Warm up properly before and cool down after your workout to prevent further strain.

- Listen to your body and stop any exercise that aggravates your pain. Consider seeking guidance from a physical therapist specializing in postpartum back pain.

Remember:

- These are general guidelines, and it's crucial to consult your healthcare professional before starting any new exercise program, especially after childbirth.

- Listen to your body, modify exercises as needed, and prioritize healing over pushing yourself too hard.

- Celebrate your progress, enjoy the process, and don't hesitate to seek professional guidance for specific concerns.

With proper modifications and a focus on gentle exercise and recovery, you can safely and effectively improve your fitness and well-being during the postpartum period.

GLOSSARY OF PILATES TERMS

Abdominal Pull: Exercise that engages the abdominal muscles while pulling the navel inward and up towards the spine.

Adduction: Movement of a body part towards the midline.

Alignment: Maintaining proper posture and positioning of the body during exercises for optimal benefit and injury prevention.

Anteversion: Tilting the pelvis forward.

Arcing: Fluid movement of the spine in different directions while maintaining a strong core.

Articulation: Controlled movement of a joint.

Balance Point: Center of gravity located just below the navel. Maintaining focus on this point helps stabilize the body.

Barrels: Half-cylindrical apparatus used for stretching, strengthening, and balance exercises.

Breathing: Deep and controlled diaphragmatic breathing, coordinating inhale with expansion and exhale with contraction.

C-Curve: Gentle rounding of the spine, similar to the letter "C."

Cadillac: Reformer-like apparatus with straps, springs, and bars for a variety of exercises.

Centering: Finding and engaging the core muscles, the powerhouse of the body.

Contraction: Shortening of a muscle to create tension and movement.

Controlled Release: Slow and deliberate lengthening of a muscle after contraction.

Footwork: Precise and coordinated movements of the feet to maintain balance and initiate movement.

Imprinting: Pressing the body into the apparatus for deep stabilization and awareness.

Neutral Pelvis: Aligning the pelvis in a level position, neither tilted forward nor backward.

Neutral Spine: Maintaining a natural curve in the spine without slouching or rounding excessively.

Pelvic Tuck: Engaging the core to draw the navel inward and tilt the pelvis slightly under.

Plantar Flexion: Pointing the toes down, flexing the ankle joint.

Post-Lateral Breathing: Advanced breathing technique where the ribs expand outwards and laterally.

Prone: Lying flat on the stomach.

Retraction: Pulling a body part back towards the spine.

Rotation: Turning the body around a central axis.

Scapula: Shoulder blade.

Scooping: Engaging the core and pelvic floor muscles to pull the navel inwards and upwards.

Supine: Lying flat on the back.

Suspension: Using the straps or springs of the apparatus to support the body and create different levels of challenge.

Teaser: Pilates exercise that requires full body coordination and control to balance on your forearms and toes.

Tucked Chin: Gently tucking the chin in towards the chest to lengthen the back of the neck.

Unwinding: Releasing tension and gradually lengthening the muscles after exercise.

This is not an exhaustive list, but it covers some of the most common terms used in Pilates. Remember that terminology and variations can differ

between different instructors and
studios.

Feel free to ask your instructor for
clarification on any terms you
encounter during your Pilates journey!